Chicken Soup for the Soul

Healthy Living:

Arthritis

Chicken Soup for the Soul
Healthy Living:
Arthritis

Jack Canfield

Mark Victor Hansen

David Pisetsky, M.D., Ph.D.

CHIEF, DIVISION OF RHEUMATOLOGY AND IMMUNOLOGY
DUKE UNIVERSITY MEDICAL CENTER

Health Communications, Inc.
Deerfield Beach, Florida

www.hcibooks.com
www.chickensoup.com

We would like to acknowledge the many publishers and individuals who granted us permission to reprint the cited material.

Aqua Angels. Reprinted by permission of Carolyn Dodge Adams. ©2006 Carolyn Dodge Adams.

A Visit from Arthur. Reprinted by permission of Lawrence Elliott. ©2006 Lawrence Elliott.

Ice Dream. Reprinted by permission of Linda Hanson. ©2004 Linda Hanson.

I Still Wear Red Lipstick. Reprinted by permission of Abha Iyengar. ©2006 Abha Iyengar.

(Continued on page 133)

Library of Congress Cataloging-in-Publication Data
is available from the Library of Congress

©2006 Jack Canfield and Mark Victor Hansen
ISBN 0-7573-0524-5

Publisher: Health Communications, Inc.
          3201 S.W. 15th Street
          Deerfield Beach, FL 33442–8190

Cover design by Larissa Hise Henoch
Inside book design by Lawna Patterson Oldfield
Inside book formatting by Dawn Von Strolley Grove

Contents

Introduction vii

The Gift of Receiving Cindy La Ferle..1
    Learning to Live with Arthritis
    What Is Arthritis?
    Think about . . . my arthritis attitude
    Treatments for Arthritis
    Think about . . . what to tell the doctor
    Children and Arthritis

I Still Wear Red Lipstick Abha Iyengar......................................27
    Dealing with Arthritis Pain
    Think about . . . positive thinking
    Think about . . . describing my pain

Ice Dream Linda Hanson 35
    Nondrug Treatments

Yoga Grandma Eileen Valinoti, R.N. 41
    Alternative Therapies
    Think about . . . alternative treatments
    Think about . . . easing my arthritis pain
    Other Health Concerns
    Working with Your Health-Care Team

Aqua Angels Carolyn Dodge Adams.............................62
Arthritis and Exercise
Think about . . . my exercise goals
Just Do It!
Think about . . . my exercise plan
Eating Right for Arthritis
Think about . . . improving my diet

Mr. Negativity Pamela Jenkins 83
Seek Support
Reduce Stress
Arthritis at Home
Think about . . . making chores easier

A Visit from Arthur Lawrence D. Elliott 103
Arthritis and Your Family
Think about . . . talking honestly about arthritis
Working with Arthritis
Think about . . . working smarter with arthritis

The Bag Lady Dances Fran McNabb.........................116
Gardening with Arthritis
Traveling with Arthritis
Think about . . . planning my trip

Resources...127
The Arthritis Foundation 128
Who Is . . . ? 129
Contributors 132

Introduction

Arthritis is one of the most common of all medical conditions but nevertheless among the most misunderstood. This misunderstanding can have important consequences for patients: delay in seeking medical attention; utilization of unproven remedies; and an attitude of discouragement, believing that arthritis is inevitable and untreatable. In writing this book, my hope has been to clear up some of this confusion and to describe the new approaches to therapy that can be of great benefit.

When I see a new patient with arthritis in my clinic, one of my very main priorities is to provide education about this condition. First, I explain what arthritis is and emphasize that there are over one hundred different diseases that have arthritis as a part. Next, I outline to the patient a plan for diagnosis. Sometimes, establishing a diagnosis is not easy because the same symptoms—joint pain and swelling—are common to all one hundred of the different diseases. Nevertheless, with a complete history and physical exam and selected X-ray and blood tests, I usually have a good idea of the diagnosis.

With a clear diagnosis, my next job is to explain to the patient the treatment options so that together we can develop a treatment plan that is right for their arthritis. The past decade has witnessed a revolution in treatment of rheumatoid arthritis, with five new and more effective drugs approved for use in this disease. The development of a single drug for a disease is remarkable. The development of five in this short period of time is unprecedented, and, indeed, can be called miraculous. With these new drugs, the outcome of treatment promises to be even brighter as physicians are raising their expectations as they strive to not only reduce symptoms of disease but even induce remission.

Not everyone with arthritis has rheumatoid arthritis. In fact, most have a condition called degenerative arthritis or osteoarthritis. For this disease, progress in treatment has also been impressive but, for osteoarthritis, the developments have been in the realm of surgery not medication. Joint replacement remains one of the most successful and beneficial of all types of surgery, with new techniques allowing replacement joints that function well for decades. I forever marvel as patients (as well as friends and family) undergo a transformation after joint replacement surgery as they switch from discouraged, tired and hurting people into vibrant and energetic people who are anxious to get on with life and enjoy activity pain-free.

This book bolsters what I as a physician can do in the clinic and provides information for how to live better with arthritis. Whatever the form of arthritis, pain is present. A physician can do only so much to reduce pain. The rest must come from the patient. Hopefully, this book will provide you with guidance, understanding and information to take charge of your disease and work better with your physician to live as happy and pain-free a life as possible.

—David Pisetsky, M.D., Ph.D.

The Gift of Receiving

Several years ago, when I was diagnosed with severe osteoarthritis in both hips, I read every book, magazine and medical pamphlet I could find about coping with chronic illness. I was amazed at how often I'd stumble on a paragraph that advised patients to "look for the gift in your pain."

Pain is a gift? Thanks, but no thanks, I'd mutter to myself. I had just turned forty-four and hadn't planned on slowing down so soon. I still had miles to go with my journalism career and a family that included a very active teenager. If pain was my gift, well, where was the return policy? Within a year of my diagnosis, the disease progressed so quickly that total hip replacement surgery was my only option.

By that time, I was unable to walk without assistive devices. Even on a good day, it hurt so much to crawl out of bed that I refused to unplug my heating pad and leave the house. Suddenly I was certifiably disabled—even qualified for a "handicapped" parking permit. Having been fit and active most of my adult life, I was way too proud to let others watch me struggle on a walker. I hated to appear needy. I didn't want pity. So I started canceling lunch dates and appointments, and tried to hide behind a steely mask of self-sufficiency.

But my closest friends and family members didn't buy any of it. And it was through their patience and love that I finally discovered the "gift" in chronic illness: It slowly unravels your pride and opens you to the boundless generosity of other people.

Of course, stubborn self-reliance isn't the sole province of the disabled. Most women I know pride themselves on being nurturers, fixers, problem-solvers, givers. We'll supply all the brownies for the bake sale at school after we've organized the rummage sale at church. We'll rearrange our schedules to babysit other people's kids. Just ask, and we'll triple our workload at the office and still make it to the evening PTA meeting. Yet some of us would rather have a wisdom tooth pulled than ask somebody else for a favor when we need it. As a girlfriend told me recently, "It's my job to be the glue that holds everyone and everything together. I can't ask for help."

The truth is, people who care about us really do want to help—if only we'd drop the facade of total self-reliance and admit that we're not all-powerful all the time.

Discussing the aftermath of September 11 and the cleanup at Ground Zero, a talk show host suggested that if anything positive rose from the ashes of the tragedy, it was that America quickly evolved from a "Me" nation into a "We" nation. As she explained it, even the most self-absorbed among us realized that we cannot function as individual islands. We need each other. It was a good lesson for me to review so soon after my first hip replacement surgery. Strapped to a hospital bed and hooked to several tubes, including an IV, I was hit with the sobering reality that I wasn't going anywhere by myself.

And during the early weeks of my recovery, I had no choice but to graciously accept support from my family and friends. When my husband processed mountains of laundry at home, I tried not to feel guilty. When our neighbors sent casseroles or offered to drive my carpool shift to school, I swallowed my pride and allowed their care to work like a healing balm. And it did. As hard as it was to surrender, I discovered there's real strength in vulnerability.

Deep down, I still believe it's more blessed to give than to receive. And I still believe that putting the needs of others first isn't such a bad precept to live by—unless it renders you incapable of accepting a favor or asking for help when you really need it. Nobody climbs her mountain alone.

♥ *Cindy La Ferle*

Learning to Live with Arthritis

If you have arthritis, you're certainly not alone. Nearly 70 million Americans have arthritis or a related condition. There are over 100 different forms of this condition that differ in severity and course. Whatever the form of disease, people with arthritis face many challenges. But the good news is that there are many ways to meet these challenges and lead a happy, healthy and fulfilling life.

Today, there are very effective therapies for certain forms of arthritis. It is easier than ever to control arthritis through the use of new drugs, surgery, exercise, joint protection techniques and creative ideas for making everyday life easier.

To live successfully with arthritis, learn as much as you can about your disease and treatment options. Work with your doctor to develop a treatment plan—and stick with it.

Yes, medications play a key role in managing arthritis. But there is much that you can do— control your weight, eat a healthy diet, exercise, reduce stress, plan your daily activities carefully— to live life to the fullest. You can control arthritis —don't let it control you!

What Is Arthritis?

When many people hear the word "arthritis," they think of aches and pains. But arthritis is much more than pain, and it is not just a disease of older adults.

The one thing that all types of arthritis have in common is that they all affect the joints—the place where two or more bones meet. Most forms of arthritis are associated with inflammation, the body's response to injury. As a result, a joint with arthritis can be tender, swollen and red. Some kinds of arthritis go beyond the joints and affect other parts of the body, including the internal organs.

These are the most common types of arthritis:

Osteoarthritis is the most common form of arthritis, affecting nearly 21 million Americans. This disease causes changes in the bone and cartilage of the joints. These changes lead to pain, stiffness, swelling and limitation in the use of your joints.

Osteoarthritis strikes most often in the knees, hips, lower back and neck, the small joints of the fingers, and the base of the thumb. Osteoarthritis tends to appear as people grow older (usually over fifty years of age) and affects women more than men. In some patients, a joint injury or misalignment increases the likelihood for osteoarthritis.

Rheumatoid arthritis (RA) affects 2.1 million Americans. RA can affect anyone, including children, but 70 percent of people with RA are women. The disease usually appears between thirty and fifty years of age. People with rheumatoid arthritis have inflammation of the lining of the joints. This inflammation can lead to long-term joint damage, including the breakdown of the cartilage and adjacent bone. This breakdown is called erosion. Rheumatoid arthritis can start in any joint, but it most often begins in the small joints of the fingers, hands and wrists. Usually if a joint hurts on the left hand, the same joint will hurt on the right hand. In most patients with rheumatoid arthritis, many joints are affected, both large and small.

The body's immune system plays an important role in rheumatoid arthritis. In a healthy immune system, white blood cells produce antibodies that protect the body against foreign substances. People who have RA have an immune system that mistakes the body's healthy tissue for a foreign invader and attacks it. This attacks leads to inflammation in the joint and erosion of cartilage and bone.

Other types of arthritis include:

- **Gout**, which affects mostly men. Gout is usually the result of an abnormality in body chemistry that leads to the formation of crystals of a substance called monosodium urate. This painful condition most often attacks a single joint, with the big toe and knee common places. Attacks can resolve by themselves but anti-inflammatory drugs can hasten recovery. Fortunately, gout usually can be well controlled with medication and changes in diet.

- **Ankylosing spondylitis**, a type of arthritis that affects the spine. This disease primarily affects men and develops when they are between twenty and forty years of age. As a result of inflammation, the bones of the spine grow together, causing stiffness and limitation of movement.

- **Juvenile arthritis**, a general term for all types of arthritis that occur in children. The course of each of these diseases differs. Some children develop rheumatoid arthritis or ankylosing spondylitis when young, while others develop types of arthritis that predominantly occur in children.

- **Systemic lupus erythematosus (lupus)**, a potentially serious disorder that can inflame joints and other tissues and affect organs throughout the body. For reasons that aren't clear, lupus develops when the immune system attacks the body's own tissues and organs. Lupus is called an autoimmune disease.

- **Scleroderma**, a disease that can cause thickening, hardening or tightening of the skin, blood vessels and internal organs.
- **Fibromyalgia**, a syndrome of widespread pain that is primarily felt in the muscles. It affects mostly women. Sometimes, fibromyalgia occurs by itself and sometimes it is associated with another form of arthritis. Fibromyalgia can also be associated with other symptoms, such as headache and fatigue.

Think about . . .
my arthritis attitude

These are the things arthritis keeps me from doing: _____

_____

_____

_____

I wish I didn't have arthritis because: _____

_____

_____

_____

If I was never bothered by arthritis, I would: ___

_____

_____

_____

Something I've learned from having arthritis is:

_____

_____

_____

Diagnosing Arthritis

To find out if you have arthritis and what type you may have, the doctor will begin by taking your medical history, doing a physical exam and performing blood tests. You may have X-rays to confirm the diagnosis, rule out other causes of pain and determine the extent of the joint damage. If your joint is swollen, the doctor may also perform a procedure called a joint aspiration, in which fluid is drained for examination.

Treatments for Arthritis

No matter what kind of arthritis you have, your doctor is likely to recommend medication for you. The type of medication that is recommended depends on what kind of arthritis you have, which is why proper diagnosis is so important.

A person with osteoarthritis may be prescribed drugs to relieve pain, while a person with rheumatoid arthritis may receive drugs that relieve pain and inflammation as well as slow down the disease process and limit further damage to joints.

Common types of arthritis drugs include:

Analgesics. These drugs ease pain that can interfere with daily activities, disrupt sleep and reduce your quality of life. They reduce pain but do not reduce the inflammation or swelling that can be associated with some forms of arthritis. The most common analgesic is acetaminophen (Tylenol). If acetaminophen doesn't ease the pain of arthritis, the doctor might prescribe an NSAID (see next entry). Other options are medicines containing opioid analgesics, such as codeine or hydrocodone, with or without acetaminophen. Tramadol (Ultram) is another widely used analgesic that has opioid properties although it may have other effects in the brain to reduce pain.

Nonsteroidal anti-inflammatory drugs (NSAIDs). NSAIDs reduce pain as well as inflammation, including swelling. Some NSAIDs—aspirin, ibuprofen and naproxen—are available without a prescription. Others require a prescription. The most common side effect is an upset stomach. Some NSAIDs, called COX-2 inhibitors, have been in the news because two of these drugs—Vioxx and Bextra—were removed from the market due to concerns over certain side effects, including cardiovascular disease. NSAIDs come with a risk of stomach bleeding and cardiovascular disease (see box on page 16, "Should You Take NSAIDs?").

Corticosteroids, such as prednisone and cortisone, are prescribed to reduce severe pain and inflammation. These prescription drugs may be given in pill form (for rheumatoid arthritis) or by injection into the joint and surrounding tissues, such as the bursae, which are structures that help keep joint motion smooth. Joint injections can only be given a few times in one year because they may weaken cartilage. Because prednisone pills have many side effects when taken on a chronic basis, doctors try to keep the dose as low as possible for the shortest time possible to keep symptoms under control.

Disease-modifying antirheumatic drugs (DMARDS) are a group of drugs that slow down the disease and limit joint damage in rheumatoid arthritis and some other types of inflammatory arthritis by reducing or modifying the body's overactive immune system. These drugs, available by prescription only, include methotrexate, sulfasalazine, azathioprine, leflunomide (Arava) and hydroxychloroquine.

Biologics are types of DMARDs that include etanercept (Enbrel), infliximab (Remicade), adalimumab (Humira), abatacept (Orencia) and rituximab (Rituxan). They help reduce pain and inflammation in RA and related diseases and are usually prescribed for people who have not found relief from other DMARDs. Biologics are proteins and must be given by injection either into a vein or under the skin. For those biologics that are given under the skin, the patient does the injection himself or herself at home. People on these medications learn to give these injections just the way someone with diabetes injects insulin. Biologics given by vein are usually administered in a specialized center so that the infusion can be supervised and side effects treated.

ARTHRITIS MEDICATION DRUG CHART

Name of medication   Dose   When I take it

_____   ____   _____

_____   ____   _____

_____   ____   _____

_____   ____   _____

_____   ____   _____

_____   ____   _____

_____   ____   _____

For each medicine, you should know:

- How to take your medicine
- How quickly it should work
- How you will feel after you take it
- When to call your doctor if you don't feel better
- Possible side effects of the medicine
- Other medicines you should not take with this medicine

Should You Take NSAIDs?

While this question is still being studied, it appears that all NSAIDs may come with at least some risk of cardiovascular disease such as a heart attack. The extent of this risk likely varies for each patient depending on age, the presence of other risk factors such as smoking or high blood pressure, as well as the dose and duration of therapy. If you're taking one of these drugs, you and your doctor have to take into account your risk of heart disease and stomach problems (ulcers or bleeding) when deciding what pain relievers are best for you.

A traditional NSAID such as ibuprofen (Advil, Motrin) or naproxen (Aleve, Naprosyn) might be a good option for people without an increased risk for heart attacks who are younger than sixty, don't have a history of stomach problems and aren't taking a blood thinner or oral steroid.

People older than sixty who have had ulcers or stomach bleeding, or take a blood thinner or oral steroid, might be steered toward a traditional NSAID plus a stomach-protecting proton pump inhibiting drug, such as Nexium, Prevacid or Prilosec. There are many factors to consider, such as other health issues, like diabetes, and if you're a smoker, so discuss your options carefully with your doctor.

Surgery for Arthritis

Surgery can be very successful for many people with arthritis. Surgery can be used to repair, replace, fuse or even remove joints damaged by arthritis. Types of surgery for arthritis include:

- **Arthroscopic surgery.** The surgeon views and repairs tissues inside your joint through small openings in the skin using an instrument called an arthroscope. Arthroscopy allows faster recovery than a procedure that opens the joint, although it is useful only for certain procedures such as repair of torn cartilage.

- **Synovectomy.** The diseased lining of the joint—the synovium—is removed to help relieve pain and swelling. This surgery can be done using an arthroscope or through traditional open surgery.
- **Joint replacement.** Damaged joints are replaced with artificial joints to relieve pain and restore joint motion and function. Joint replacement is most commonly performed for large joints such as the hip or knee. These are major procedures that may require considerable time for recuperation and rehabilitation.
- **Fusion.** Adjacent bones at a joint are fused or joined together to eliminate the motion that causes pain or increases instability of the joint. Joints in the spine are frequently fused.

If your doctor recommends surgery for your arthritis, here are some questions to ask:

- What other kinds of treatments could I have instead of surgery? How successful might those treatments be?
- How long does this surgery usually take?
- What are the risks involved? How likely are they?
- Can the surgery be done on an outpatient basis?
- Am I likely to need a blood transfusion? Will I have to donate my own blood?
- How much improvement can I expect after the surgery?
- Will I need to go to a rehabilitation facility?
- What kind of assistive device, such as a cane or walker, will help me?
- How long will I need to use one of these devices?

- What help will I need at home with activities such as bathing or getting out of bed?
- Will more surgery be necessary? After how long?
- What happens if I delay surgery?
- Do I have to stop any medications before surgery?
- Can you give me the name of someone else who has had this type of surgery?

Signs Your Arthritis May Be Getting Worse

If you answer "yes" to any of these questions, it's time to discuss your treatment with your doctor. These signs may indicate you need a change in treatment.

Yes	No	
_____	_____	I finish a bottle of pain medicine faster than I used to.
_____	_____	I spend a lot of time in bed, aside from my regular sleep time.

Yes   No

_____   _____   I drink alcohol to ease my pain.

_____   _____   I talk about my pain or arthritis much of the time.

🌳 Think about . . .
what to tell the doctor

Before you go to the doctor, think about these points so you're ready to discuss them.

My pain started:_____

My pain feels like: _____

My pain lasts for:_____

My pain is worst at this time of day:_____

The pain affects the joints in these parts of my body: _____

Things that make my pain better or worse:_____

_____

Medications that have eased the pain:_____

_____

Other symptoms I've noticed:_____

_____

Other medical conditions I have: _____

_____

Childhood illnesses I've had:_____

_____

Adult illnesses I've had: _____

_____

Joint surgeries I've had: _____

_____

Injuries I've had: _____

_____

Lifestyle habits (such as smoking, drinking or exercise): _____

_____

Medical conditions my family members have had: _____

_____

Children and Arthritis

Childhood arthritis is actually a group of diseases. As a group, these diseases are called juvenile rheumatoid arthritis (JRA) although only some children with this condition actually have rheumatoid arthritis. Children can have inflammatory diseases that resemble those that occur in adults while there are certain forms of arthritis that appear to occur almost only in children. To try to reduce confusion, some physicians call this group of diseases JIA for juvenile idiopathic arthritis. In some children, JRA or JIA is a self-limited condition that affects only a few joints and eventually goes away. But other children suffer joint and tissue damage from JRA as well as slowing of growth, causing short stature.

Children with JRA may have inflamed, stiff or bent joints. They may have joint stiffness after they rest or slow down, and weakness in muscles and other tissues around the joints. They may not want to exercise or do regular physical activity. Some children with JRA develop eye inflammations or other eye problems. JRA affects each child differently, and it may affect the same child differently on different days.

Treatment for children usually includes medication, exercise, eye care, dental care and healthy

eating. Because children are still growing, treatment of their arthritis must be done with great care
and usually is best accomplished by a specialist.

Helping Your Child Cope with Arthritis

If your child is diagnosed with arthritis, he or
she may feel angry or sad. They may blame you.
They may also resent siblings who don't have
arthritis.

You may feel a range of emotions as well, from
sadness to anger to guilt. But it's important to
remember that your child's arthritis is not something you could have prevented.

To help your child:

- Talk about their feelings, and yours. Allow your
  child to express their anger, sadness or confusion.
- Let your child know you still have high aspira-
  tions for them. Help them set goals and
  encourage them to participate in activities that
  they are physically able to do.
- Learn as much as you can about the disease
  and its treatment, and help your child to learn
  as much as possible, too. Talk with teens about
  the importance of sticking to their medication
  regimen to prevent flare-ups and to prevent
  complications in the future.
- Try not to be overprotective—help your child
  find out what tasks they are capable of doing.

- Talk to your child's teachers, school nurse and principal about arthritis and its effects on your child. A member of your child's health-care team may be able to provide information for school staff.
- It's especially important for the gym teacher to understand your child's condition. Children with JRA need to pace themselves in gym and participate in gym activities that do not hurt involved joints.

I Still Wear Red Lipstick

Time was when, as an agile girl, I thought nothing of skipping rope or jumping in the air to catch that ball. Marriage and babies made a sitting spectator out of me. Over the years, weight collected around those once well-toned muscles while I sat happily with the babies, books, computer and cherry pie.

With the kids grown up and in college, I decided to resume a more active life. It began with taking frequent walks in the nearby park. And so I was introduced to creaking knees and painful joints and subsequently, to help me, an orthopedist.

After studying the X-rays of my knees and hipbone, the orthopedist fixed me with his bleary eye. I fluttered haplessly like a butterfly on a pin board, awaiting his verdict.

"You have osteoarthritis setting in," he said grimly. "You are also overweight, and your bones are protesting. You want to keep walking the rest of your living years?" I nodded, my head down, feeling like a child caught playing truant. "Then you better start walking now. . ." He said this quietly, seriousness writ large on his face.

I had tried walking in the park, I told him. That's how I realized things were not as they should be. My hip, knees, calves and the soles of my feet ached alternately, simultaneously, or in unison when I walked. I hated walking.

". . . to be able to walk," he reiterated.

He then fixed me with his second bleary eye. "You are overweight." Second statement, second nod.

"Your knees cannot support the extra load. You have to lose weight, say, twenty pounds. Change your diet—remove white bread, white rice, white sugar from it completely."

He sure did hate white. "What do you drink? Milk?" My answer would make him happy. "I love black coffee. I drink lots of it!" I said triumphantly.

"Have lots of milk to strengthen your bones. Plus a calcium supplement." He did not approve of black coffee and was advising milk. It wasn't color after all.

I found his gaze straying to my legs. I crossed them delicately, to show off my pointed, high-heeled pumps. These were my favorites, with silver buckles for extra pizzazz. It was only natural that I preened a bit.

He looked disapprovingly at my well-shod feet. "Fine varicose veins like spiders up the back of your legs—that's what overweight and high heels bring about. With arthritis setting in, high heels are highly avoidable." For me, this consultation was becoming highly avoidable. My face turned beet-root red, a color that had no effect on him.

"Please, then, no high heels. I would advise you wear Dr. Scholls, which is sensible footwear. It will help your aching legs."

He did not care about my aching heart. The only things that made me feel glamorous nowadays were that dash of color on my lips and my high heels. I felt all-woman when I wore my lipstick and my heels. I could give up black coffee, but my black pumps? This man did not know the first thing about female psychology.

"Now remember, diet, walking, milk, no high heels—these changes are essential. Most impor-tant, you are carrying excess baggage, and your legs are buckling under this. Lose weight or you will lose all. I don't care how you do it. Join a gym or exercise on your own, whatever you do, the answer lies in getting into shape."

I, the pinned, fluttering, hapless butterfly was finally released from the doctor's unflinching gaze. He handed me my X-rays, his prescription and a fat bill.

I told myself I would never visit him again. The only way to do this, unfortunately, was to follow his advice. With angry tears coursing down my cheeks, I threw my heels away. I then went and bought the brightest of red lipsticks in defiance.

My husband returned home to see me wearing my new, hot lip color. He played it safe. "You look good," he said. He knew all about my psychology.

After a while, he asked, "How did it go?"

"I've thrown away my heels. It's supposed to make some of the pain go away, but that hasn't happened yet," I sobbed in frustration and despair.

It took me some time to lose my weight, but I was determined to get my body working again. The aches and pains in my joints have reduced, and I feel more energized and alive. Walking is something that I do every day.

No more fat or fat doctor bills, just fresh air, fruits and Dr. Scholls! I'll say cheers to that, with a bright smile on my hot-red lips. A woman can't give everything up.

♥ *Abha Iyengar*

Dealing with Arthritis Pain

Arthritis pain can be caused or worsened by several factors, including:

- Inflammation, which causes the tenderness, redness and swelling in your joints.
- Damage to joint tissues, which results from the disease process or from stress, injury or pressure on the joints.
- Fatigue that comes from having arthritis, which can make your pain seem worse and harder to handle.
- Depression or stress, which can come from limits on your activities, including doing the things you enjoy. Some new studies indicate that getting the inflammation caused by arthritis under control can bring depression under control, too.

Ways to Control the Pain

With so many treatments for arthritis now available, many people who in the past might have had to settle for a life of pain now can live comfortably. If you're experiencing regular pain, don't just accept it as an expected part of your disease. Talk to your doctor about what other treatments you could try.

If you still experience pain despite medications that your doctor can prescribe for you, here are some ways to try to make the best of it:

Ask what your body is telling you. Try thinking about the message your pain is sending you. For instance, is it telling you that you've been sitting too long?

Find alternatives. When you're feeling well, come up with a list of things to think about or do to try to take your mind off the pain when it does come.

Think positively. Concentrate on positive self-talk instead of negative messages. Instead of telling yourself you're too tired to exercise, come up with reasons why you'll feel better after you do exercise—such as you'll sleep better. Negative messages can lead to increased pain, while positive messages can help distract you from pain.

🌳 *Think about . . .*
positive thinking

Here are some negative self-talk statements I've made in the last two days:

1) _____

_____

2) _____

_____

3) _____

_____

Here's how I can change those negative statements into positive ones:

1) _____

_____

2) _____

_____

3) _____

_____

🌳 *Think about . . .*
describing my pain

Here are some things to discuss with my doctor.

My pain is located:_____

_____

_____

_____

During the past month, I have had to cut down on my time at work (arriving late or leaving early) _____ days because of my arthritis pain.

I've had to limit my activities, such as moving a table, writing, sewing, playing a musical instrument, pushing a vacuum cleaner, hammering, bowling or playing golf:

__ A lot
__ A little
__ Not at all

Ice Dream

I grew up in Wisconsin. Ice skating was my favorite winter activity. Playing crack the whip with cold wind blasting against my face allowed me to feel the reckless abandon of speed we often seek as children.

When I was hospitalized for knee pain at nineteen I was diagnosed with arthritis. I was shocked. In my twenties, along with visits to an obstetrician, then a pediatrician, I visited a rheumatologist. I started to think I'd never be able to play actively with my children, never take them ice skating. I was advised to give up my bike, volleyball and stairs. My skates hung in the garage on a nail, unused. One day they were given away.

By thirty-five, I had started my third type of medication to handle the disease when my husband's job moved our family south. The warm weather eased my joint pain. I was able to discontinue all prescribed medication. When my children had skating parties with their school, I enjoyed renting skates. I loved taking the hands of small

children on ice for their first time, helping them
around their circular path. When one little girl I
helped remarked that I must be an Olympian, my
husband was quick to remind me it came from a
six-year-old girl. He supported my activity, though,
by giving me passes to the ice rink for gifts. I often
asked my coworkers to skate with me instead of
meeting for lunch.

But after a fifteen-year reprieve my husband was
told he had to transfer back to the Midwest or lose
his position. Dreading the return to cold weather, I
anticipated finding a new rheumatologist. After we
settled, I found work in a rehabilitation setting.
Part of my job is to encourage patients with serious
breathing problems to exercise. It felt fraudulent to
push others, some using oxygen tanks, when I was
not an example myself.

I began going to a gym early mornings before
work. Initially my treadmill walks took almost
thirty minutes for one mile. I was afraid of further
knee problems. Despite occasional nights when the
pain in my knee prevented me from a quick pas-
sage into sleep, I persisted.

Now I walk three times a week at a pace of four
miles an hour. I walk an entire hour, increasing the
speed at intervals depending on what beat is com-
ing through my headphones. I have been back
in cold weather for two winters and remain off

prescribed medication. I'm able to be an example to the patients I encourage to take their first steps on the treadmill. I can't say I'm totally pain-free. There are nights I lie in bed with intense knee pain. But on those rare occasions, I use relaxation techniques I teach to my patients. My focus is to keep moving.

Last winter for my fiftieth birthday my husband took me to Rockefeller Center in New York City. With the Christmas tree lit, the holiday music playing, the crowd above, we held hands and ice-skated. We didn't play crack the whip, but once again I felt free gliding on that ice. My ice dream came true. Now I wonder, could I try hockey?

♥ *Linda Hanson*

Nondrug Treatments

There are a number of nondrug treatments you can try to lessen the discomfort from arthritis. They can be as simple as an ice pack, a heating pad, a massage or a warm bath.

Heat and Cold

Using heat and cold treatments can ease the pain and stiffness of arthritis. Heat relaxes your muscles and stimulates your blood circulation. Try dry heat—heating pads or heat lamps—as well as moist heat—warm baths or heated wash cloths. Cold packs make sore areas numb, and reduce swelling and inflammation.

Here's how to make the most of hot and cold treatments:

- Use a towel between your skin and the hot or cold pack.
- Use heat or cold for only 15 to 20 minutes at a time.
- Use an electric blanket or mattress pad in the morning before you get out of bed to help ease morning stiffness.
- Try a warm shower in the morning to reduce stiffness.

- To prevent burns, turn off your heating pad before you go to sleep.
- Check with your doctor before using cold packs if you have poor circulation.

Massage

Many people with arthritis report that massage makes them feel better by bringing warmth and relaxation to the painful area. You can ask your doctor to recommend a professional who is trained to give massages (you'll want to check with the massage therapist to make sure they have experience working with people who have arthritis).

You can also massage yourself. Here are some pointers:

- Don't massage a joint that is very swollen or painful.
- Use lotion or oil to help your hands glide over your skin.
- Use firm, gentle strokes and pressure, especially over your joints where skin and muscle layers are thin. If you press too hard you could irritate the joint or muscle you are trying to help.

Water Therapy

Soaking in a warm tub doesn't just feel good—it's actually good for you, too. You may want to install rails to make it safer and easier to get in and out of the tub. If you have trouble with the tub, try a warm shower. Applying heat can relax muscles and decrease pain and stiffness. Taking a warm bath gets heat to many parts of your body all at once.

You may also find it's easier to move in warm water, so exercise becomes easier. Try doing gentle exercises in the tub or warm shower in the morning to get you moving. Taking a warm bath before bedtime can help ease pain that's built up during the day, and help you sleep.

Yoga Grandma

It had been a hectic day in the emergency room where I worked as a registered nurse. All day long we were run off our feet dealing with patients with heart attacks, victims of automobile accidents or injured children needing sutures. At day's end, I eased into the front seat of my car looking forward to going out to dinner with friends. But when I put my foot on the gas pedal, I felt a sharp pain that radiated from my groin down my right leg. At first I thought the pain was from the constant running up and down on the hard-tiled floor of the emergency room, but in the following days, even when I was off, the pain persisted. Soon I found myself hobbling instead of walking at my usual brisk pace.

"You have arthritis in your right hip," the doctor said after examining me and checking my X-rays. Arthritis! I was stunned. No one in my family had it, and at forty-eight, I considered myself young. I swallowed hard, trying not to show how upset I felt.

The doctor patted my arm reassuringly.

"You have to stay positive," he said. "Keep active without putting too much stress on the joints and come back to see me in six months."

I made up my mind not to let arthritis take over my life, but as the weeks passed, I could no longer keep up the hectic pace in the emergency room, racing on winged feet from one crisis to another.

"You need to apply for a job with less physical stress," my supervisor told me gently one day. My heart sank; I loved my work in the emergency room, priding myself on my quicksilver reactions. "Faster than a speeding bullet," my coworkers had joked. But, I realized, that was in the past.

"I know there is a nursing vacancy in the geriatric clinic," she went on. "Why don't you apply?" She put a hand on mine, seeing tears well in my eyes.

But I knew I had to face reality, so I said a sad good-bye to my friends in the emergency room, and the following week, I applied for and was hired in the geriatric clinic. Many of the elderly patients there were arthritis sufferers, and I felt a new empathy with them I hadn't had when I was bursting with good health. Who was I to complain, I thought. I could still hold down a job and get around. In contrast, many of my patients needed canes or walkers or even wheelchairs. Still, most of them were cheerful, even jocular. I stopped feeling sorry for myself, inspired by their example.

For the next year, my arthritis remained at bay. I enrolled in a low-impact exercise class, walked every day after work and swam in the local pool. But then, all at once, the pain in my hip flared. Putting weight on my right leg was extremely painful. I had to take a leave of absence from work and go to the hospital for physical therapy every day.

I found myself staying at home after the physical therapy sessions, a heating pad wrapped around my waist, glued to the TV and getting up only for snacks. Soon I was gaining weight and feeling depressed. It was a dreary winter, and as I looked out the window, my mood would become as gloomy as the threatening skies. I worried, too, about my daughter. She was expecting her first baby in the spring, and I had promised to help her. But now, our roles were becoming reversed. She was calling daily to see how I was and had started doing my grocery shopping for me. I felt that I had lost control of my life.

Then, one day, a flyer from the local YWCA came in the mail.

"Therapeutic yoga classes will begin next week—perfect for arthritis sufferers and for the aches and pains of life," the notice read.

"Yoga"—the word brought to mind chanting in incense-scented rooms, willowy types in black leotards in exotic poses, white-robed swamis. Could this class possibly be for me? "Why don't you try it, Mom?" my daughter said when I told her about it. "What do you have to lose?"

Nothing at all, I thought. I had to get out of my rut, which was turning into a deep, dark hole. So with my doctor's permission, I enrolled in the class. On a sunny Monday morning, I found myself in a classroom at the Y with several other ladies who were busy laying out their mats on the floor. A cheerful young woman with dark, smiling eyes introduced herself.

"I'm Daisy, your teacher," she said. "Welcome to our therapeutic yoga." Then she lowered the blinds and put on a CD, instructing us to lie down on our mats, close our eyes and begin just by "observing our breathing." Next she guided us through the "wave breath," a breath beginning in the upper chest and ending in the belly.

"Put your hand on your belly and feel it expand like a balloon," she said.

As I breathed deeply and listened to the soothing music that filled the room, I felt my stresses melt away. Then Daisy took us through gentle stretching, putting all the joints through easy range-of-motion exercises, while at the same time telling us to concentrate on our breathing. I felt the tension leaving my muscles and my mind clearing as I focused on "the breath." I left the class feeling energized, and as I walked out to my car, a new hope rose in my heart.

The class met three times a week, and the more I practiced, the more limber I felt. The stiffness and even the pain in my joints diminished. Soon I abandoned my heating pad and my spot on the couch and once again did my own grocery shopping. I felt a new confidence that arthritis need not take over my life.

When I went back to work, the patients and my coworkers exclaimed, "You look wonderful. What have you been doing?"

"Therapeutic yoga," I answered. I could tell by their baffled expressions that they had the same misunderstandings that I had had.

"I don't stand on my head," I said laughing. When I explained that therapeutic yoga was simply gentle exercise and stretching and deep, relaxing breathing, they understood.

On a gorgeous spring day, my daughter gave birth to a beautiful baby boy, my first grandchild. Each day I climbed the stairs up to her fifth floor walk-up apartment to help her care for the baby. One lovely afternoon we put the baby in his carriage and took him for a walk. As we strolled together in the park, the budding trees and flowers seemed to be celebrating this new, precious life. I felt reborn, too, in my new role as grandmother.

Yoga is a Sanskrit word meaning "union" or "yoke" or "to harness together." As I walked with my daughter and the baby, I thought about how therapeutic yoga helped me to keep connected, not only with my classmates as we bent and stretched together, but with my daughter and now my precious grandson.

♥ *Eileen Valinoti, R.N.*

Alternative Therapies

There are many so-called alternative therapies advertised for arthritis. Many people who use these therapies don't tell their doctor because they're sure the doctor will disapprove, or even stop treating them. Some of these therapies are pills, while others are devices such as copper bracelets or magnets.

It's important to consider that a treatment that's strong enough to help you could also be strong enough to harm you. All of these alternative therapies may have side effects. That's why you should tell your doctor about any herbal remedies or nutritional supplements you're taking in addition to over-the-counter or prescription medicines.

These alternative therapies are not regulated by the government, so there is much that isn't known about them, such as the proper dose and how they may interact with other alternative or approved treatments. Also, these therapies do not have to meet the same standards of purity as conventional drugs, leading to uncertainty about safety and side effects.

If your arthritis pain isn't being adequately controlled by conventional medicine, it can be very tempting to try an herb or supplement that promises to ease your pain.

If you are considering one of these products, ask

your doctor, pharmacist or other health-care professional whether they think it is safe and could help your type of arthritis. Since these therapies are not approved, however, they are not covered by insurance. The costs for alternative therapy can easily mount, and if you're on a budget, you may want to consider whether this is the best way to spend your money.

Glucosamine and Chondroitin Sulfate

These popular supplements are sold under many brand names and can be found in capsules, tablets, liquid or powder. Glucosamine is made from the shells of shrimp, lobsters and/or crab, and chondroitin is made from the windpipes of cattle or pork by-products.

Past studies show that some people with mild to moderate osteoarthritis taking either glucosamine or chondroitin sulfate reported pain relief at a level similar to that provided by NSAIDs such as aspirin and ibuprofen. Some research indicates that the supplements might also slow cartilage damage in people with osteoarthritis.

Findings from a major study called the Glucosamine/ Chondroitin Arthritis Intervention Trial were published in early 2006 in the *New England Journal of Medicine*. This study of people with osteoarthritis in the knee found that glucosamine and chondroitin were no better than a placebo (fake pill) in reducing knee pain in the majority of patients. But it did find that the combination of the two supplements provided significant pain relief for the group of people with moderate-to-severe knee osteoarthritis. The results of this study have been controversial since it is not clear why this therapy should work only in this group of patients.

Based on the findings from this study, the Arthritis Foundation recommends that people with knee osteoarthritis speak to their doctors about whether combined glucosamine-chondroitin therapy might be a beneficial addition to their overall treatment plans.

Words of Caution

Some people should not take glucosamine/chondroitin or should be especially cautious if they do:

- Children, women who are pregnant and women who could become pregnant shouldn't take these supplements because they have not been studied long enough to determine their effects on a child or developing fetus.
- People with diabetes who take glucosamine should check their blood sugar levels more often since this supplement is a type of sugar.

- People who are taking chondroitin plus a blood-thinning medicine or daily aspirin should have their blood clotting time checked more often. Since chondroitin is similar in structure to a common blood-thinning drug, the combination may cause bleeding in some people.

Hands-on Therapies

There are a number of hands-on treatments for pain relief in addition to massage. These include:

Chiropractic. Chiropractic care involves the manipulation and manual adjustment of the spine. Manipulation of some joints may help relieve pain from osteoarthritis, but joint manipulation of weak or damaged joints could cause problems. Tell your chiropractor that you have osteoarthritis and make sure he or she has experience working with people with arthritis.

Acupuncture and Acupressure. These ancient Chinese pain-relief treatments are gaining popularity in the United States. In acupuncture, needles are used to stimulate specific points throughout the body. In acupressure, practitioners use their fingers instead of needles. If you choose one of these therapies, make sure your practitioner is licensed and certified.

🌳 *Think about . . .*
alternative treatments

These are alternative treatments I've tried: _____

_____

_____

This is what I thought about their effectiveness:

_____

_____

Alternative treatments I'm considering trying are:

_____

_____

Here's what I need to find out about them first:

_____

_____

🌳 Think about . . .
easing my arthritis pain

Here's what I've used at home to treat my arthritis pain and how well they worked:

Treatment	Very Effective	Somewhat Effective	Not Effective
1)_____	☐	☐	☐
_____			
2)_____	☐	☐	☐
_____			
3)_____	☐	☐	☐
_____			
4)_____	☐	☐	☐
_____			
5)_____	☐	☐	☐
_____			

Other Health Concerns

Osteoporosis

A common problem for people with arthritis is the loss of bone tissue, causing a condition called osteoporosis. Osteoporosis occurs more commonly in women than men and increases as people grow older. In osteoporosis, if too much bone is lost, bones become weak and can break easily. Such fractures occur commonly in the spine and cause a loss of height as well as a bent or crooked back. Your doctor can find out if you have osteoporosis or are at risk for fractures in the future through a painless and noninvasive test called a bone mineral density test.

You can lower your risk of bone loss and osteoporosis by making changes to your lifestyle:

Do regular weight-bearing exercise. Try doing 30 minutes a day of physical activity, such as walking, on most days. Choose something you like to do. Check with your doctor before beginning any exercise program.

Get lots of calcium. You need calcium for building and maintaining healthy bones. Women (and men) age fifty-one and older should get 1,200 milligrams of calcium a day. Calcium-rich foods include low-fat milk and cheese, and broccoli. Foods that may be fortified with calcium include orange juice, cereals and breakfast bars. If you can't get enough calcium from the foods you eat, you may need to take a calcium supplement.

Don't forget vitamin D. Your body needs vitamin D to absorb calcium. If you don't get enough vitamin D, you won't be able to absorb calcium from the foods you eat, and your body will have to take calcium from your bones. The recommended amount of vitamin D is 600 to 800 IU per day. Good food sources of vitamin D are fortified dairy products, egg yolks, saltwater fish and liver.

Ask your doctor if you should be taking medication to prevent bone loss. There are medications both to prevent and treat bone loss due to osteoporosis. The most common of these drugs are called bisphosphonates. Fosamax (alendronate), Actonel (risedronate) and Boniva (ibandronate) are bisphosphonates. These drugs deposit in the bone itself and reduce a process called resorption that is part of a cycle of turnover in which bone is resorbed, or carried away, and is then built back. Other drugs for osteoporosis include estrogens, SERMs (selective estrogen receptor modifiers) and parathyroid hormone. The use of estrogens is controversial because of the risk of breast cancer and ovarian cancer in women.

Don't smoke, and if you drink, do it sparingly.
Smoking increases your risk of osteoporosis, and
drinking alcohol increases your risk of falling and
breaking a bone.

Heart Disease

Recent research has shown a link between the
inflammation involved in arthritis and an increased risk of heart disease. For conditions such as
rheumatoid arthritis, there is evidence that the
treatments that reduce the inflammation in arthritis may also reduce the likelihood of heart disease.
This evidence points to the importance of proper
diagnosis and treatment and the use of effective
medications to lower the amount of inflammation
in disease. To further reduce risks to your heart, the
following steps are important:

- Don't smoke.
- Have your blood pressure, blood glucose and
  cholesterol levels checked regularly.
- Eat less saturated fat and more fruits, vegetables, grains, low-fat or nonfat dairy products,
  fish, beans, poultry and lean meats. Reduce the
  amount of salt and alcohol you consume.
- Exercise regularly (see the chapter in this book
  on exercising with arthritis).
- Watch your weight. Aim for a body mass index

(BMI), a measure of body fat based on height and weight, between 18.5 and 24.9 and a waist measurement of no more than 35 inches for women and 40 inches for men. To calculate your BMI, go to *www.nhlbisupport.com/bmi/ bmicalc.htm.*

Working with Your
Health-Care Team

A person with arthritis often deals with many health professionals. You will usually start with your main health-care practitioner—such as your primary care physician, internist, or in the case of children, pediatrician. Some of the other health-care workers often involved in arthritis care include:

- **Rheumatologists** specialize in the treatment of people with arthritis or related diseases that affect the joints, muscles and bones. You may be referred to a rheumatologist if you need special care or treatment. All rheumatologists are internists who have had extra training in the care of people with arthritis and related diseases. For certain forms of arthritis, such as rheumatoid arthritis, rheumatologists have a very important role in treatment because of their experience in diagnosis, their understanding of the many different drugs that are used and their ability to administer drugs such as the biologics that require intravenous infusions.

- **Pediatric rheumatologists** specialize in treating children with arthritis or related diseases through the teen years.

- **Orthopedic surgeons** specialize in the treatment of musculoskeletal conditions and may be consulted to perform certain surgical procedures to help in diagnosis as well as repair joints if they are damaged.
- **Physiatrists** are medical specialists who can direct your physical therapy and rehabilitation.
- **Podiatrists** are experts in foot care. If arthritis affects your feet, a podiatrist can prescribe special supports and shoes for you. Podiatrists also may perform surgery to correct foot deformities.
- **Occupational therapists** can teach you how to reduce strain on your joints while doing everyday activities. They can fit you with splints and other devices to help reduce stress on your joints.
- **Physical therapists** can show you exercises to help keep your muscles strong and your joints from becoming stiff. They can help you learn how to modify your home and use special equipment so living with arthritis is easier.

When you visit a doctor, it can help to bring along a list of your medications as well as the bottles themselves to make sure that you have all the right medications and are taking them correctly. This is especially true if you are on a variety of different pills. It may help to have a friend or relative come with you. You can talk with that person about what happened during the visit and compare notes.

Don't be afraid to ask the doctor questions and request clear explanations about your arthritis and your treatment program. You may want to write down these questions to make sure that you do not forget anything important.

Questions you may want to ask include:

- What can I do to decrease my pain?
- What are the risks and benefits of treatment?
- How will the treatment affect my other health problems?
- How much will the treatment you are recommending cost?
- Are there less expensive options such as generic (non-brand-name) drugs?
- Which arthritis symptoms are to be expected, and which ones should I call you about?
- Can you provide me with written materi brochures or suggest a reliable source of mation on the Internet?
- Are there any programs in the com can help me with my arthritis?

Getting a Second Opinion

It's important for you to fee medical care and your in

doctor and the doctor's staff. There are times, however, when you may be uncertain or unhappy about your care, or you may not like the style or personality of a particular doctor. Don't dismiss those feelings—you may have a long-term relationship with the people treating your arthritis, and if you don't feel at ease talking with one of them, you may want to consider switching doctors.

Or you may not feel comfortable with your doctor's recommendations. In that case, you should think about getting a second opinion. Another specialist might have a different perspective on arthritis treatment and give you new information.

Here are some tips on how to get a second opinion:

- Ask your doctor to recommend a specialist for
  ... opinion. Don't worry about hurting
  ... feelings. You may be able to get a
  ... friend or colleague, or
  ... tis Foundation
  ... hritis.org).
  ... ysicians by

  ... e provider to
  ... d opinion, and
  ... ing to is covered
  ... ou need a referral
  ... tor.

- Have your doctor send medical records to the doctor you're seeing for a second opinion, so you don't have to repeat any medical tests. Your doctor's office may charge a fee for this service.
- As with your regular doctor, come prepared to meet the new doctor with a list of questions and concerns.
- Ask this doctor to send a written report to your regular doctor, and get a copy for your own records.

Aqua Angels

I was diagnosed with juvenile rheumatoid arthritis when I was just three years old. For my entire life I have heard the words, "but, you are too young to have arthritis," and unfortunately, these words have not been true. . . .

I painfully remember being a child with arthritis during grammar school. I was embarrassed by my body, had difficulty moving and never really felt free. I think the hardest part was feeling so different from my classmates. It is hard enough to be a kid, but when the simplest tasks like sitting cross-legged on the floor become a moment of anxiety, body image and shame take on a whole new childhood meaning.

When you are a child, you are not supposed to think so much about every move you make. You are not supposed to have pain as you struggle to walk across the playground. And you are not supposed to feel so trapped within your own fear. Unfortunately, when you are a child with arthritis, these feelings take center stage, and you are forced to grow up quickly.

I was lucky. I had wonderful, supportive parents and friends who wanted me to feel included and normal and encouraged me to participate in many activities. Even with all the love and support, I still felt trapped within my own stiff, painful, swollen joints. So often I just wanted to escape—to not feel every step and movement, to feel free to run and play like other kids. But that just wasn't my reality.

During high school my arthritis took a real turn for the worse. I was in the middle of a terrible flare-up with the disease, and it just wasn't getting better. On the worse days, I remember not being able to raise my own arms to brush my hair. This limitation was extremely daunting to a sixteen-year-old girl. Some days it was hard to just get out of bed, get out of a chair or dress myself. I felt that I was a sixteen-year-old girl trapped in a ninety-year-old body.

During this time I became more depressed and much more embarrassed by my body. It didn't help that I had gained so much weight—weighing more than 200 pounds. I know that some of this weight gain was due to the medications, but most of it was due to my lack of activity. I moved less and less, became heavier and heavier, and more and more depressed.

Both of my parents are amazing athletes, which sometimes made me feel that much more like a failure. But my parents are also wonderful models of encouragement. My mother saw what was happening to her sixteen-year-old daughter—the isolation, the weight gain, the depression—and she decided to sign me up for an Arthritis Foundation Aquatic Class. I, of course, did not want to attend. I certainly did not want anyone to see me in a bathing suit. But as usual my mother won out, and I joined the Arthritis Foundation Aquatic Program.

I was sixteen, and the ladies in the pool were seventy years and older. They wore their skirted bathing suits and their pink-flowered bathing caps. They were named Wertebell, Ethel and Maybel, and I will tell you that these amazing aqua gals changed my life.

While I could hardly get into the pool because of the stiffness and pain in my joints, they flew past me. While I could hardly do one repetition of an exercise, they could do ten. But when I entered the pool nothing mattered but finding joy in how much I could move. My wonderful aqua gals encouraged and supported me. I remember, for the first time in my life, feeling like I could do something to help my body. I remember feeling hope. But most important, I remember feeling pride. I felt as though I was on to something; that maybe, just maybe, life wasn't over and I wasn't alone.

Those aqua classes and those aqua gals changed my life in more ways than I can ever express. With time, I slowly found grace and power of movement in a body that had always embarrassed me. And that feeling is one that has stayed with me through all of the good days and bad with arthritis.

Today, twenty years after I stepped into my first aqua class, I find myself a trainer for the Arthritis Foundation. I have taught and trained more instructors to carry on the message of hope and inspiration that my wonderful aqua angels taught me. Every time I step into the pool I say a little "thank you" to them. For I know that they watch me in their pink-flowered bathing caps and skirted suits. I know that they encourage me to keep moving even on the days that it is so hard. And I know that they believe in me, and through them, I belong.

♥ *Carolyn Dodge Adams*

Arthritis and Exercise

Exercise, when done properly, can help a person with arthritis in many ways. Exercise:

- keeps your joints flexible
- keeps the muscles around your joints strong
- helps strengthen bones
- improves your ability to do daily activities
- improves your overall health and fitness by:

  —giving you more energy
  —helping you sleep better
  —controlling your weight
  —making your heart stronger
  —decreasing depression
  —improving your self-esteem and sense of well-being

Getting Started

The best exercise program for you depends on the type of arthritis you have, how severe it is and which joints are affected. Even if your arthritis has affected your feet, knees or hips, you still can enjoy exercise with a program that won't aggravate these joints. Consult your doctor before starting any exercise program to make sure that it is appropriate for you and will not stress your heart, for example. Your doctor can refer you to one of these specialists who can help you design a program that's right for you:

A **physical therapist** can show you special range-of-motion and strengthening exercises to help keep your joints flexible and your bones and muscles strong. They also can teach you proper exercise techniques, precautions and other guidelines.

An **occupational therapist** can show you how to do everyday activities in ways that won't place additional stress on your joints. Occupational therapists also can provide you with splints or other assistive devices that can help you exercise more comfortably and reduce pain.

There are three types of exercise that are recommended for people with arthritis. They are:

Range-of-motion exercises. These exercises reduce stiffness and help keep your joints flexible. The "range of motion" is the normal amount your joints can be moved in various directions. These exercises should be done every day. Examples of range-of-motion exercises can be found on the Arthritis Foundation Web site at *www.arthritis.org*, or by ordering their brochure, *Exercise and Your Arthritis*, by calling 800-283-7800.

Strengthening exercises. These exercises help maintain or increase muscle strength. Strong muscles help keep your joints stable and protected. These exercises also should be done every day.

Strengthening exercises include both isometric exercises (in which you tighten your muscles but don't move your joints) and isotonic exercises (in which you move your joints through a range of motion to strengthen muscles against some form of resistance). Consult your doctor, a physical therapist or occupational therapist about how to do these exercises.

Endurance exercises. Once you feel comfortable doing strengthening and range-of-motion exercises, gradually start endurance exercises (such as walking and water exercises). This type of exercise will give you more stamina, so you can go longer without getting tired as easily. It will also help you sleep better, control your weight and feel better overall.

Start small—five minutes, three times a day. Slowly expand from 15 minutes a day total to 30 minutes, most days of the week.

Walking

All you need to start walking is a good pair of supportive walking shoes. If you have severe hip, knee, ankle or foot problems, talk to your doctor; you may want to skip the walking and do your exercise in a pool.

Water Exercise

Swimming and exercise in warm water are especially good for stiff, sore joints. Warm water (between 83°F and 88°F) helps relax your muscles and reduce pain. Water helps support your body, so there is less stress on your hips, knees, feet and spine. You can do warm-water exercises while standing in shoulder- or chest-height water or while sitting in shallow water. In deeper water, use an inflatable tube or flotation vest to keep you afloat while you exercise.

Bicycling

You can improve your fitness through bicycling, especially on an indoor, stationary bike. Adjust the seat height so that your knee maintains a slight bend when the pedal is at the lowest point. Don't add so much resistance that you have trouble pedaling. Start slowly, and if you have knee problems use little or no resistance.

Tips for Exercising Safely

- Exercise during the time of the day when you are feeling less pain and stiffness and when you have adequate time to exercise.

- Don't do strenuous exercises just after you eat or just before you go to bed. Wait at least two hours after a meal.
- Exercise on a regular basis. Try to do range-of-motion exercises daily and your strengthening and endurance exercises every other day.
- If you miss a day, pick up again where you left off. If you miss several days, you may need to start again at a lower level.
- Warm up before exercise and cool down afterwards for 5 to 15 minutes to reduce the risk of injury.
- Wear loose clothing and comfortable shoes with good support. The soles should be made from nonslip, shock-absorbent material.
- Take your time. Exercise at a comfortable, steady pace. If you can't speak to someone without running out of breath, you're going too fast!
- Stop exercising right away if you have chest pain or tightness, have severe shortness of breath, or feel dizzy, faint or sick to your stomach. Contact your doctor immediately.
- If you develop muscle pain or a cramp, gently rub and stretch the muscle. When the pain is gone, continue exercising with slow, easy movements.
- If you have some discomfort in your joints

following exercise, you may want to reduce the type of exercise or the intensity. If a joint stays inflamed or painful after exercise, you may want to consult your doctor to determine whether you should continue the program.

🌳 Think about . . .
my exercise goals

My long-term exercise goal is to: _____

_____

My short-term steps for getting to my goal are:

1)_____

_____

2)_____

_____

3)_____

_____

Family members and friends I will ask to help
and to provide feedback on how I'm doing are:

1)_____

2)_____

3)_____

Just Do It!

There will be days when you just don't feel like exercising. Do a little less on those days, but if a joint is inflamed or tender, it may be best to wait until symptoms subside.

Here are some ways to resist your negative self-talk about exercise:

"It's boring." Choose exercises you enjoy. Do different types of exercise on different days to mix it up. Listen to upbeat music while you're exercising. Exercise with friends or family members.

"I don't have enough time." Make a schedule and stick to it. It's okay to exercise for several short periods instead of one longer period. Remember, this is special time that you're making for yourself.

"The weather's bad." If you can't get to the gym or pool, exercise at home that day. If you usually walk or swim outside, walk inside a mall on a rainy day.

"I don't like to exercise alone." Ask friends or family members to exercise with you or join an exercise class.

Yoga and Tai Chi

These ancient practices are gaining popularity among people with arthritis.

Yoga consists of balancing exercises and gentle stretches that condition the entire body. Doing yoga every day can improve your flexibility and balance and increase muscle control. It is also a great way to relax. Some types of yoga are more strenuous than others. You'll want to find an instructor who is familiar with arthritis and the limitations it can impose.

Tai chi is an ancient Chinese practice designed to exercise body, mind and spirit. Tai chi improves balance and may be able to reduce the risk of falling, which is an important benefit for someone with fragile bones and joints. Start with a class—a teacher can make sure you are doing the movements correctly. Once you learn the basic moves, you can practice on your own or with a video.

🌳 *Think about . . .*
my exercise plan

FITNESS CONTRACT FORM

Week of: _____

This week I will: _____

_____

What type of exercise: _____

_____

How much: _____

When: _____

How many days: _____

How certain I am: _____

(On a scale from 0–10, with 0 being totally unsure and 10 being totally confirmed. Note that ideally, a person should achieve a level 7 certainty.)

SIGNATURE: _____

Eating Right for Arthritis

There are many reasons to eat a healthy diet when you have arthritis. Perhaps the most important is that controlling your weight will help you lose extra pounds that are hard on your weight-bearing joints in the hips, knees, back and feet. Of course, a healthy diet may also reduce your risk of heart disease, diabetes and cancer. And it will make you feel better.

To eat a healthy diet, follow these guidelines:

- **Eat a variety of foods**—breads and grains, fruits, vegetables, dairy products, and meats. Variety will ensure you are getting all the nutrients your body needs.
- **Use fat and cholesterol in moderation.** To follow a diet low in saturated fat and cholesterol, choose low-fat cuts of meat, such as poultry or flank steak; use nonfat or low-fat dairy products; and limit amounts of fats, oils, salad dressings and sweets.
- **Eat plenty of vegetables, fruits and whole-grain products.** They're usually low in fat and high in fiber, which can help you lose weight.
- **Use sugar and salt in moderation.** Check the sugar content of the foods you eat. Look on food labels for the words dextrose, sucrose,

fructose, honey, corn syrup solids, dextrine and maltadextrine—these indicate added sugar. A lot of processed foods, such as canned soups, packaged sauces and gravies, pickles, prepared frozen dinners, restaurant fast foods, and tomato products, are high in salt. Some arthritis drugs, such as prednisone and NSAIDs, also may increase the amount of sodium in your body. Sodium causes your body to retain water, which can affect your blood pressure.

- **Drink alcohol in moderation.** Too much alcohol can weaken your bones, which can lead to osteoporosis. Alcohol also leads to weight gain, since it adds extra calories to your diet. Alcohol doesn't mix well with certain arthritis medications. For instance, stomach problems are more likely if you combine alcohol with aspirin or other nonsteroidal anti-inflammatory drugs (NSAIDs). Large amounts of alcohol combined with acetaminophen or methotrexate can cause liver damage. Alcohol also can increase uric acid in the blood and aggravate gout. If you are taking any medications for arthritis you should check with your doctor about drinking alcohol, even in moderation.

Keep Track of What You're Eating

Many of us eat more than we think . . . or are willing to admit. One way to know for sure just what you eat in a typical day is to keep a food diary, like this one:

Food Diary

Food or Drink						
How much	What kind	Time	Where	Alone or with whom	Activity	Mood

This type of food diary also can help you make connections between the types of food you eat and why you eat certain things. For instance, do you eat more when you're alone? Then try to be around other people when the urge to eat strikes. Do you tend to eat a lot when you're lonely or grumpy? Make a list of nonfood alternatives that you can turn to when you're feeling low.

Arthritis-Food Connection?

While there is no "arthritis diet," there are some connections between food, nutritional supplements, and certain forms of arthritis and their related conditions:

Gout. A type of arthritis, gout is caused by deposits of monosodium urate crystals in the body. Monosodium urate forms from a substance in the blood called uric acid, which is a breakdown product from cells. Alcohol and foods such as organ meats, legumes, sardines and anchovies, and broths and gravies can contribute to levels of uric acid and the tendency to gout. When you have gout, your body either has trouble getting rid of uric acid or your body produces too much uric acid, which forms the crystals. Medications, combined with a diet that limits meats, legumes (dried beans, soybeans and peas), sardines and anchovies, broths and gravies, and alcohol, can reduce uric acid levels in people with gout.

Osteoporosis. People with rheumatoid arthritis, juvenile rheumatoid arthritis or lupus are at risk of developing osteoporosis, a condition in which the bones weaken and tend to fracture (see "Other Health Concerns" on page 53 for more information on eating right to reduce your osteoporosis risk). Osteoporosis develops more readily when the diet is low in calcium.

Beware of Unproven Diet Claims

Those diets, foods and supplements that come with a claim that they can cure arthritis are too good to be true. Most of these products have not been scientifically tested to determine if they're safe. In fact, some of these diets may even have harmful side effects, including those that include large doses of alfalfa, copper salts or zinc, or the so-called immune power diet or the low-calorie/low-fat/low-protein diet.

Food Preparation Tips

Having arthritis can make meal preparation a challenge. Joint pain, swelling, limited mobility and fatigue can all work against you in the kitchen. Here are some tips to simplify cooking:

- Plan rest breaks while you're preparing meals.
- Think about how your kitchen is arranged—

are the utensils you use the most in a place where they're easy to reach? If not, consider rearranging things.

- Use labor-saving kitchen gadgets and appliances, such as electric can openers and microwave ovens.
- Look for kitchen tools that have large, comfortable grips.
- Sit on a high stool while cooking or washing dishes.
- Use a small, soft-grip pair of needle-nose pliers to pull open small tabs and seals on jars.
- Buy healthy "convenience" foods at the grocery store, such as pre-sliced or chopped vegetables, or already-cooked grilled chicken tenders.
- Add fresh fruit and whole-grain bread to a frozen dinner to make a complete, satisfying meal.

Think about . . .
improving my diet

Ways I can improve the way I eat:

1) _____

   _____

2) _____

   _____

3) _____

   _____

4) _____

   _____

5) _____

   _____

Mr. Negativity

I heard about Bill several months before I actually met him. He was a hot topic of conversation in the doctor's office where I took treatments for rheumatoid arthritis. The nurses were afraid of him, and the other RA patients tried to avoid his company. This wasn't easy to do, as the treatments lasted about three hours. Like it or not, once a patient was settled in a chair and the potent medication in the IV drip bag was flowing, there weren't a lot of options.

Usually I was able to share a small room with other patients during the visit. The nurses, office manager and doctors were in and out of our room during the course of the treatment. There was a friendly atmosphere of laughter and conversation. Some patients were nervous about being pricked with a needle, so this helped them to relax. Coffee and cookies were offered, and friendships were made. We all had one common bond. We hurt and ached, and we were seeking relief from the pain.

My first clue that all was not well in the office

came when a flustered young nurse stopped outside the door to my room. I overheard her ask a
male nurse to please take over one of her patients.
She just couldn't go back into Bill's room again. I
couldn't help but wonder why, and it piqued my
curiosity. Who was Bill?

Some of the other patients had already met Bill.
"He's quite an old curmudgeon," one whispered to
me. Another said, "He made our nurse cry. He was
rude to her." There were rumors that instead of coffee, he would ask for a shot of bourbon. When one
nurse told him she was going to give him an injection, he growled, "Well, I'll drop my pants and
moon you, but only if you moon me back."

Bill's medication did not seem to be giving him
the relief from pain that was expected. He was
quick to tell other patients, especially the new
ones, that the treatments were worthless and they
shouldn't waste their money. He liked to remind
them of the side effects, scaring one young woman
into almost canceling her dose. While the other
patients tried to reassure her, our nurse murmured,
"I just don't know what we're going to do about
Mr. Negativity."

When the morning came that I finally met the
infamous Bill, I was surprised. I was expecting
someone rough and intimidating. What I saw was
a frail old man who walked with careful, shuffling

steps. He was dressed well and his silver hair neatly combed. He stopped and stared at me before sitting down in the vacant chair next to mine. I braced myself for the assault I was sure to come.

"Hello, I'm Bill. How are you doing today?" he asked politely. "You takin' this stuff, too? I'll bet by tonight you'll be the best dancer at the ball. Doesn't seem to help me much, though." At this point one of the nurses stepped forward and began to prepare Bill for his injection. He sighed deeply, and I realized that the medical staff was running interference for the rest of us, keeping Bill from bothering the patients around him.

I saw a grimace of pain on Bill's face as he settled himself into a more comfortable position. The scowl should have been a warning to others that he wanted to be left alone, but my heart began to ache for the pain I knew Bill was feeling.

I made up my mind then to spend a little time getting to know Bill. A chronic illness can make a person feel isolated and alone. I could tell he was lonely and was probably depressed about his lack of progress with the medication. I had been in that position myself a few times over the years, and I understood firsthand how frustrating it could be. It was probably hard for someone like Bill to start a conversation with those around him when the primary thing on his mind was his health.

It didn't take much effort to change the subject from our aches and pains to our other interests. Before long, Bill and I were talking about our jobs, families, church activities and life in general. As Bill began to open up, I noticed other patients listening. He became more animated, and his blue eyes sparkled with mischief. One of the nurses pulled up an office chair and sat mesmerized by the tales of his younger days. The office manager soon joined us as we laughed at the idea of Bill pulling off pranks as a child. The other patients were smiling, too. Our morning was definitely looking brighter.

At the end of my visit, with the IV removed and the Band-Aid in place, I was ready to leave for the day. I turned to Bill and said, "It's been very nice to meet you, Bill. I've enjoyed visiting with you today."

Bill smiled in return, and thanked me for spending a little time with a grumpy old man. Then he added, "And you know, I think I'm going to be feeling a lot better this time around."

I believe I will, too, Bill. In fact, I feel better already.

♥ *Pamela Jenkins*

Seek Support

One of the most difficult aspects of having a chronic illness like arthritis can be the feeling of losing control over one's health. A person with arthritis may find themselves staying at home more, which can increase loneliness and stress.

By becoming part of a support group, participants can gain a sense of control over their disease. They get out of the house and meet other people and become motivated to take action. They start to feel better both psychologically and physically.

Participants often pick up valuable tips and techniques from fellow arthritis patients. Sharing stories and advice can help group members feel good about themselves and stay motivated to maintain and improve their health.

Finding you're not alone with invisible but very real pain is another important plus of support groups. No matter how supportive family and friends are, they don't know exactly how you feel—that's why having "arthritis friends" is so helpful.

Is a Support Group Right for You?

- Do you like being part of a group?
- Do you like to talk about your feelings with others?

- Do you want to hear stories about other people and their arthritis experiences?
- Are you looking for helpful hints, or do you want to share your advice?
- Would such a group make you feel better?

To find an arthritis support group:

- Call your local Arthritis Foundation office and ask for a list of support groups in your area, or view listings online at *www.arthritis.org*.
- Ask your doctor for recommendations.
- Call your local hospital to see if they have a group.
- If you can't find a support group in your area or you have a hard time getting out of the house, look for an Internet support group for people with arthritis.

Reduce Stress

Here's a great reason to try to relax: stress can actually make pain worse. Stress can even cause pain in some cases.

A person with arthritis may have a lot to be stressed about. You might be spending a lot of energy thinking about your pain. Friends and family members may not understand what it's like to have arthritis and fail to offer enough support. And having arthritis can make activities at work and at home more difficult.

Stress can take many forms, from snapping at someone without meaning to, to suffering from headaches, an upset stomach, muscle tension or teeth grinding. Stress can also lead you to unhealthy and dangerous habits, such as smoking or drinking.

Identifying Stress in Your Life

Think about the stress in your life. Ask yourself what causes it and how you respond to it.

One effective way to answer these questions is by keeping a stress diary. This can help you identify stressors that may not always be obvious to you, and help you link your physical and emotional reactions to certain types of stress.

Stress Diary

Date	Time	Cause of stress	Physical symptoms	Emotional symptoms

Once you identify what causes your stress and how you react to it, then you can begin to develop coping strategies so that in the future you'll deal with stress more effectively.

Sometimes, just knowing what causes your stress isn't enough to help you deal with it. If you feel that your stress is taking over your life, or if you feel depressed, consult a mental health professional. There are many effective treatments, including medication, counseling and psychotherapy.

Learning to Relax

Strange as it sounds, you may have to learn to relax if you've become accustomed to stress as a way of life. True relaxation will bring your heartbeat and temperature back to normal, untense your muscles and reduce pain.

There are many ways to relax your body and mind:

Guided imagery helps you focus on pleasant images. Begin by breathing slowly and deeply. Think of yourself in a place where you feel comfortable, safe and relaxed. Imagine the colors, sounds, smells and feelings. These images take your mind off of your pain and focus it on something more enjoyable.

Prayer can be very relaxing and comforting for

some people. You may want to make a tape record-
ing of a soothing inspirational message or practice
your own personal prayer.

Hypnosis is a form of deep relaxation and
guided imagery. You'll need to work with a professional psychologist, counselor or social worker
who is trained in hypnosis. You can also learn self-
hypnosis techniques that you can practice on your
own.

Relaxation audiotapes and DVDs/videotapes
provide directions for relaxation, so you don't have
to recall the instructions. You can make your own
tape of your favorite relaxation routine.

De-Stress Your Life

Say no. It's hard to do, but you need to prevent
yourself from getting overbooked so you have some
time to yourself.

Ask for help. Make yourself delegate at home
and at work. People may not do things just the way
you want them to, or as fast as you'd like. But at
least you won't be doing everything yourself.

Learn to compromise. Get used to not having
your house perfectly clean all the time. The differ-
ence between "very clean" and "pretty clean" isn't
big enough to worry over.

Get moving. When you feel that familiar stressed-
out feeling, go for a walk, or do some yoga.

Work with your boss. Would a more flexible schedule make life easier for you? If you've been at your job for a while, your boss may be willing to work with you to make your hours more manageable—perhaps you can get in earlier and leave earlier to avoid rush-hour traffic, for instance.

Keep a journal. Let it all out on paper. You may find relief from writing down your feelings.

Improve Your Sleep

If you're in pain, it can be difficult to get a good night's sleep. But being well rested is just what's needed to combat stress. Here are things you can do aside from taking a sleeping pill that can help you get that solid eight hours you're craving:

Exercise regularly. Don't do it too close to bedtime, though—some people find it stimulating.

Soak in a warm bath. You'll relax sore muscles, making sleep come more easily.

Try not to nap. You may be exhausted from a poor night's sleep, but if you nap in the afternoon, you'll just be keeping the cycle going. If your disease is very active and the level of inflammation in your body is high, a period of rest during the day can be helpful.

Skip the caffeine. Afternoon or evening caffeinated drinks can interfere with nighttime sleep.

Check your medications. Some medicines can affect your mood and your ability to get to sleep. If you think your medicine is part of the problem, ask your doctor if you can change the dose or timing of the medicine. Don't just stop taking it on your own.

Arthritis at Home

There's always at least ten things you need to do around the house. With the complications that arthritis can add to your life, it may seem like you're always behind in your chores.

The first thing to do is to set your priorities. Yes, you eventually do need to do laundry, but you can come up with ways to do it smarter. Same for cleaning, shopping and personal-care tasks. Here are some hints to get you started.

Grocery Shopping

Wear the right footwear. Cushioned shoes that support your feet will make the trip much more comfortable.

Bring a reacher for grabbing light, nonbreakable items on shelves.

Get help. Ask a family member, friend or neighbor to come with you. Either they or a salesclerk can help you get heavy items from the shelf or bend or stretch to get items that aren't in easy reach.

Call ahead. Find out if your grocery store provides delivery service, so you won't have to lug bags to and from the car. Or maybe your local store provides free bag service so someone else can unload the bags into your car.

Get organized. Make a shopping list broken down by store aisle, so you won't have to retrace your steps. Stop at the manager's desk first to ask for help with heavy items, like laundry detergent or dog food.

Take it easy at home. Don't try to put away all the groceries at once. Put away frozen and refrigerated foods first, then take a break before storing away everything else.

Cleaning

Pick arthritis-friendly tools. Use tools that won't force you to bend down, such as long-handled dustpans and a long-handled toilet brush. Clean windows using a mop with a squeegee and a long handle, and ceilings with a long-handled mop, so you won't have to overstretch.

Plan ahead. Wear a work apron with pockets so you can stash cleaning supplies such as bottles, sponges and rags. That way you'll avoid repeat trips to the closet. Don't load yourself down with too many supplies or else you'll strain your back and shoulders.

Cart it around. Get a wheeled utility cart so you can push supplies from room to room. Or get a garden cart/seat on wheels so you can sit on it as you wash lower walls or clean the bottom of cabinets, drawers and appliances. You can store cleaning supplies on the cart.

Keep multiple supplies on hand. Buy enough supplies so you can keep some in the bathrooms, kitchen, and upper and lower floors.

Use convenience products. Automatic toilet bowl cleaners, spray-on mildew removers and shower-cleaning spray will help you reduce scrubbing.

Remember to sit. Some tasks, such as polishing silver or folding clothes, can be done sitting down.

Take rest breaks. Don't do everything at once—plan breaks to help prevent overdoing it.

Protect your joints. Keep your hand flat when using a dust cloth, or use a duster that fits over the whole hand, to avoid a gripping motion that can hurt your joints. When you clean with water, use a large sponge instead of a cloth, so you can squeeze out the water easily by pressing down on the sponge with the palm of your hand.

Make it a party! Hire your grandkids or neighborhood children to come in and clean up. Give each one several tasks, and reward them—pizza and a movie, anyone?

Laundry

Color code. Buy a different-colored laundry bin for each family member, and keep it by the washing machine. When the laundry is done, sort the laundry into each person's bin, and let them carry it to their rooms themselves.

Sit and load. Get a chair to put by the washing machine, so you can sit while you load and unload the washer and dryer.

Wheel around. Use a wheeled laundry cart to collect laundry from different rooms and return it when you're done.

Have someone else do it. Even if it's too expensive to send your laundry out to be cleaned all the time, consider doing so for heavy-when-wet items such as bedspreads and curtains.

Personal Care and Dressing

- Sit on a bath stool in the shower or tub.
- Install rails to help getting in and out of the tub.
- Wash with a bath mitt, bath puff or long-handled brush.
- Use nonskid mats in the tub and shower.
- Extend or build up brush and comb handles by attaching rulers, foam rubber or pipe insulation tubing.
- Use an electric toothbrush or one with a built-up handle.
- Use a freestanding mirror to put on your makeup, so you don't have to lean over the sink and strain your back.
- Use a zipper pull or add a loop or large paper clip to make it easier to grasp the zipper.
- Look for jackets with Velcro closures.

🌳 *Think about . . .*
making chores easier

Here are strategies I want to try to make my daily routines easier:

Shopping

1) _____

_____

2) _____

_____

3) _____

_____

Cleaning

1) _____

_____

2) _____

_____

3) _____

_____

Laundry

1) _____

_____

2) _____

_____

3) _____

_____

Personal care/dressing

1) _____

_____

2) _____

_____

3) _____

_____

Protect Your Joints

As you go about your daily tasks, it's important to remember to protect your joints by using them in ways that avoid extra stress. Here are some do's and don'ts to help you.

Task	Right	Wrong
Climbing stairs	Go up by leading with stronger leg; go down leading with weaker leg.	DON'T put pressure on your weaker leg.
Lifting objects	Hold items close to your body.	DON'T put pressure on your arms, hands or back.
Opening jars	Use the palm of your hand or a jar opener.	DON'T grasp or twist your fingers.
Traveling	Divide travel items into two equal loads or use a suitcase with wheels.	DON'T carry unequal loads.

Use Assistive Devices

Canes, crutches, walkers and scooters can be a great help to people with arthritis. They reduce stress on your hips and knees. Use a cane when you go up stairs, and take advantage of scooters provided in large stores.

A Visit from Arthur

Grandma was born in Oklahoma in 1924, but she was raised in Wichita, Kansas. In the 1950s, she settled in the then up-and-coming Southern California city of San Diego. In time, she became a seamstress and a very good one, indeed. After many years in the garment business, a friend would occasionally pop into her life. Her friend was named Arthur.

Arthur was a bothersome friend who would cause her great pain in her life. Before Arthur, she could sew undisturbed for hours and hours. Some of her creations included suits, dresses, gowns and other garments. But over time, Arthur would have none of this. He was a relentless hindrance, and he would not allow her to do something she was not only good at, but also what she truly loved.

Initially, Arthur would limit her sewing to the point she couldn't do it for as long as she wanted. But as Arthur became more and more demanding, her hours spent sewing diminished. In time, she was only able to sneak in a few other activities in an attempt to fill her time with something creative.

"I'm having a visit from Arthur," she would say with a sly smile. I grew to dislike Arthur for causing her so much pain and for being such a burden on her life.

You see, Arthur was really arthritis.

Grandma never let arthritis affect the one thing she used to keep it from robbing her of her dignity: humor. She always seemed to make the darkest day seem like the sun was shining bright. She never let arthritis or anything else cripple her humor. There wasn't much she could do, she would always say, so why not make the best of it. She could always stitch humor into every dark situation, and I loved her for that.

Grandma passed away at the age of seventy-five. She lived a full life, and that's really all any of us can ask for. I'd like to think she is in heaven, sitting behind a little sewing machine, glasses hanging on the tip of her nose, without Arthur to disturb her, creating a garment for the angels. That's a nice thought.

Recently, my wife was diagnosed with osteo-arthritis in her knees. "I guess I'll be getting a visit from Arthur, too," she said with a smile. In fact, we both smiled. It made us think of Grandma.

♥ *Lawrence D. Elliott*

Arthritis and Your Family

When one person in the family has arthritis, it's everyone's business. If you have arthritis, your partner will need to accept more responsibility around the house. You may not be able to do some of the things you did as a couple or family, especially if you've done sports together or are used to being constantly on the go.

Your kids will learn that you can't necessarily run around with them or pick them up. They may have a hard time understanding why you get so tired, and they may worry that you will become bedridden or disabled. They might think they did something to make you sick.

Having arthritis can be a challenge. But if everyone in your family can learn to communicate clearly and openly about how the disease is affecting your lives, it needn't be a negative influence. In fact, having arthritis can force you to strengthen your family bonds.

Communicate. Let family members know that it's okay to express their feelings of anger, frustration or sadness about how arthritis is affecting your family. Don't let bad feelings build up and explode.

Ask for help. Don't hesitate to get the help you need from those closest to you, especially for activities that cause you pain or fatigue or put stress on your joints.

Involve the family. Get everyone's input about decisions regarding how to share chores and make new arrangements in your home that are more arthritis-friendly.

Reassure your kids. Tell them that arthritis can be properly managed and treated. Explain the basics of the disease to them so they're not confused and they understand the likely course of the disease and what problems could occur. Of course, this means that you have a clear understanding yourself. Invite their questions.

Preplan activities. You may not be able to do the family activities you used to do, but that doesn't mean you can't still have special, enjoyable times together. It just requires some preplanning on your part. Think about something your family can do together that won't place too much physical stress on a person with arthritis.

🌳 *Think about . . .*
talking honestly about arthritis

My partner and I need to talk more about how arthritis is affecting these areas of our relationship:

__ sharing household chores

__ sharing child care

__ finances

__ social life

__ sex life

__ feelings of anger or frustration

__ other _____

I'd like to talk more with my children about:

__ their feelings about having a parent with arthritis

__ how arthritis is affecting family activities

__ how they could help out around the house more

__ the facts about arthritis and its treatment

I wish I felt more comfortable talking with my
family about this issue: _____

_____

_____

_____

_____

_____

_____

_____

_____

_____

_____

_____

_____

_____

_____

_____

_____

Working with Arthritis

Arthritis can have an impact on your job, no matter where you work. From getting to work, to sitting or moving around comfortably once you get there, to deciding how to communicate with your boss and coworkers about your condition, there are many variables to consider.

You also need to be creative in finding ways to do your work without becoming exhausted or doing activities that could aggravate your arthritis. Having a positive attitude is key.

Some ways to get through your workday without worsening your aches and pains include:

Stay fresh. Make a regular bedtime schedule, and stick to it, so you get enough rest for the next day.

Commute in comfort. See if you can share a ride with someone, so you don't have to drive every day, or take turns driving. If public transportation is convenient, try to use it to give yourself a break from the hassles of driving. If you do drive, get a backrest or supportive seat for comfort.

Look closely at your work area. How can you arrange things so you can limit the amount of lifting, carrying, reaching, holding or walking that you do each day?

Vary your activities. Don't sit too long in one

position or repeat one motion too many times—
mix things up to avoid strain and injury. If your job
requires a lot of sitting, stand up every half-hour or
so, stretch and walk around.

Set your priorities. Do the most important
tasks early in the day, when you feel the strongest
and have the most energy.

Exercise. Ask your doctor if there are easy exercises you can do at work to help you—such as
bending your fingers, wrists and elbows for a few
seconds at a time.

Stay Comfortable at Work

- Sit in an adjustable chair. Your lower back
  should be against the backrest, and your feet
  should be on the floor.
- Keep your files and supplies within easy reach.
- Use devices to decrease stress on your body,
  such as document holders attached to your
  computer monitor, footrests, a wrist rest for
  your computer and armrests for your chair,
  and a hands-free telephone headset.
- If you use a computer, your upper body should
  be about 2 feet from the monitor. The top of
  the monitor should be at an even line with the
  top of your head.
- Sit close to the keyboard—it should be 3 to 6
  inches from your lap—so you don't have to

reach out for it. The monitor and keyboard should be directly in front of you, not off to the side.

Talking to Your Employer About Your Arthritis

Talking about your arthritis with your boss and coworkers can be a source of worry and concern. Once they know about your arthritis, they may question your ability to do your job. If they don't know much about arthritis, they may think you're getting special treatment or making a big fuss over nothing. This is especially true with certain forms of arthritis where there is much more pain and fatigue than would be apparent from your appearance. Some people are concerned that their arthritis will be held against them at promotion time.

However, there are some good reasons to discuss your arthritis at your workplace. Employers don't have to make changes in the workplace as required by the Americans with Disabilities Act (ADA) if they don't know about your disability. If your coworkers don't know why you get tired easily or suffer from aches and pains, they may not give you the support you may need to get through the day. And if you are trying to hide your arthritis, you may overdo it and put too much stress on your body, increasing your pain and fatigue.

Planning the Conversation

Before you talk to your employer about your arthritis, plan the conversation carefully. Ask your doctor or an occupational therapist to recommend any assistive devices or changes to your work that would ease your arthritis symptoms.

When you meet with your supervisor, describe how arthritis may affect your work. Talk about any changes you could suggest to make you more productive. Make it clear you want to make the situation work for everyone.

If you are suggesting devices to make your job easier, find out ahead of time how much they cost. Tax deductions and/or tax credits may be available to certain employers who provide accommodations and/or jobs for people with disabilities. You can find out more on the Americans with Disabilities Act Web site (*www.ada.gov*).

Telling Potential Employers

If you have arthritis that may impact your work or cause you to take off time from your job, you may be tempted to avoid telling a potential employer. But if you're hired, your employer will find out eventually—and could be disappointed or annoyed that you weren't open in the first place. Those feelings could even color your employer's view of you from that point on. It's better to be hired by someone who accepts your condition and is open to working with you to help you do your job well.

Health Insurance

Insurance coverage is very important, especially if you are on expensive medicines. If you start a new job, make sure to find out what care is covered and how to transfer your care. You want to be sure that coverage for treatment continues as you make the transition from one employer to another. The Department of Labor (*www.dol.gov*) has information on the Health Insurance Portability and Accountability Act (HIPAA), which provides rights and protections for participants and beneficiaries in group health plans. HIPAA includes protections for coverage under group health plans that limit exclusions for preexisting conditions and prohibit discrimination against employees and dependents based on their health status.

Choosing a New Job

If you're looking for a new job, think about your physical capabilities and how they match the position you're seeking. Ask yourself:

- How much standing, walking and sitting am I comfortable doing?

- How much lifting and reaching can I do?
- What is my fatigue level?
- Can I hold objects or open car doors easily?
- Can I perform repetitive hand movements without aggravating my symptoms?

When thinking about a new job, write down the activities involved and how your arthritis might affect your ability to perform each activity.

You may want to ask an occupational therapist to help you determine whether you could do a specific job comfortably, and whether any equipment or accommodations could make it easier for you to do the job.

If you cannot come up with workable solutions, you may want to start thinking about other jobs in the same field that would interest you but would be less taxing on your body.

🌳 *Think about . . .*
working smarter with arthritis

Reactions I've received to my arthritis at work are:

_____

_____

I could make my job easier on my body if I made
these changes:

1)_____

_____

2)_____

_____

3)_____

_____

Here's how I feel about discussing these changes
with my supervisor: _____

_____

_____

The Bag Lady Dances

They call me the bag lady.

No, I don't walk the streets and dig in trash cans, but I do carry a bag everywhere I go. This bag might be made of canvas or leather, but usually it's nothing more than a plastic supermarket bag. It doesn't matter as long as it's filled with shoes. I never go anywhere with only the shoes on my feet.

In 1989 when I realized I couldn't make it around the walking track or stand in front of the classroom all day, I found myself sitting in the doctor's office. After a thorough examination and blood work, my doctor recommended that I be tested for rheumatoid arthritis.

"Oh, no," I said. "There's no way I have arthritis. I'm only thirty-eight. I think I'll go to a podiatrist."

So I did. Several hundred dollars later, I found myself sitting in my doctor's office again, watching the nurse draw the blood that would show positive for RA. I was devastated because the rheumatologist I eventually got in to see wasn't very encouraging.

"It might be slow. It might be fast. You might have periods that you think it's gone, but the RA will be with you, and you will get worse."

I walked out of her office with a lump in my throat. That was fifteen years ago, and I can honestly say the words of that first rheumatologist came true. It's been a slow process, thank goodness, but the RA hasn't gone away.

My feet were the worst. Every day I walked into the classroom wearing a decent pair of shoes. By noon, I was in my second or third pair, usually a big pair of clunky walking shoes, and by the end of the day, I walked out of my classroom wearing slippers. My bag of shoes became my symbol.

Three foot surgeries and a medical retirement later, I still carry my bag of shoes, but not with as many. Since I'm off my feet most of the time now, I have graduated to one or two pairs a day, but I always have the uglies ready to put on.

I searched for months for the right pair of shoes to wear to my son's wedding. I wanted to show up in shoes like all the other ladies, but most of all I wanted to dance. Dancing had always been a joy for me, and even though my husband and I have stayed off the dance floor in recent years, I was determined to dance for this wedding.

I found a pair of shoes that matched my dress, not fancy, but okay. I had them stretched three times, filled them with pads, and walked into the wedding with them on my feet. When it came time for the mother and son dance, I swallowed, gritted my teeth and walked out onto the dance floor with my new, in-style, matching shoes that had already begun to hurt. In the middle of the dance, I couldn't go any longer. I had to stop.

Trying not to cry, I looked up to tell my son that the dance was over, but before the words came out, he whispered. "Mom, take them off so we can dance."

I nodded and gave in. Embarrassed that the entire wedding party was watching me, I tossed my shoes to the side and figured I'd just have to be the brunt of the evening's jokes. I was going to dance with my son. Instead, the room exploded in applause. How wonderful to have understanding friends and family members.

I didn't carry a bag into the wedding that night, but I had strategically placed dancing slippers under my table. The nice, matching shoes never went on my feet again.

To this day, I hate spring and summer. All my friends shop for cute little sandals while I scour the stores looking for something, anything, that I can wear. My closet is filled with shoes that I buy, wear a couple times, then discard.

Vanity can be a terrible thing—and expensive to

boot. Every time I clean out the bottom of my closet, I chuckle at the bags lined up waiting for me to stuff them with shoes, but I always take a moment to touch the satin slippers that let me dance the entire night at that wedding.

I've been called a lot of things in my lifetime. I guess "bag lady" isn't bad at all.

♥ *Fran McNabb*

Gardening with Arthritis

Gardening is a popular hobby that may not seem that arthritis-friendly. But with the right kind of tools and some advance planning, you can enjoy gardening as much as you did before you developed arthritis. And if you haven't taken up gardening, you might want to consider it!

Stretch before you start. Do gentle stretches to loosen your joints and prevent injury. One stretch to try: reach your arms straight out in front of you as far as you can.

Get the right tools. Use long-handled tools that let you stand instead of stoop. Get easy-to-grip hand tools. Find something to sit on while weeding, such as a scooter wagon or kneeling pad.

Pay attention to posture. Stand or sit up straight, and change positions often. Don't use your fingers to lift—use the flat palm of your hand instead.

Don't do it all at once. Take frequent breaks so you don't overdo it. Consider hiring someone to help you, particularly with the heavy work.

Flowerbox power. Plant in a flowerbox instead of a regular flowerbed to avoid stooping.

Traveling with Arthritis

Today there are more choices than ever for a person with arthritis who wants to travel. Not every trip may be appropriate for you, of course, but there are many destinations that will make for an enjoyable vacation, with a little advance planning.

General Travel Tips

- If you're visiting friends or family during the holidays, send packages ahead. Either buy gifts online and have them shipped, or send them yourself before you leave to avoid having to carry heavy loads.
- Consider staying at a hotel instead of with friends or relatives. If you can afford it, staying in a hotel can be more relaxing. You can get extra room, soak in a warm tub as long as you like, and avoid stair-climbing.
- Bring extra prescriptions with you (not in checked luggage that can get lost), so you can replace medication that gets lost or used up.
- Bring your doctor's name and phone number and a summary of your medical history in case of delays or emergencies.
- Pack light! If you don't have luggage with wheels, get some—your joints will thank you.

- If you need to eat with your medicine, pack a light snack—airlines have cut down on food service, and the train food service car may be a long way from your seat.

Air Travel

- If possible, book a nonstop direct flight to avoid the hassle of transferring planes.
- Ask for a seat in an exit row or just behind the bulkhead for more room.
- If you have trouble walking, ask for a wheelchair or motorized cart in advance.
- Ask skycaps to check in your luggage.
- Prevent stiffness during a flight with simple range-of-motion exercises and getting up and stretching as much as you can. Roll your shoulders and flex your ankles, hands and fingers.
- Whenever possible, walk up and down the aisle or to the restroom.
- Bring a lightweight carry-on bag to hold your medications, along with a change of underwear and socks, a toothbrush and other necessities. That way if you're stranded en route, because of bad weather or a missed connection, you won't have to worry if you don't have access to your checked luggage.

Car Travel

There are many items that can make car travel more comfortable for a person with arthritis. The types of devices that can help you depend on which parts of the body are affected, how severe your arthritis is and how long a trip you'll be taking. Ask your doctor for recommendations.

Items that some people with arthritis find helpful include:

- A horseshoe pillow for head and neck support
- A cervical collar to prevent neck pain
- A lumbar pillow for added back support
- Cushions to absorb vibrations or soften the seat for sore hips and backs
- A cushioned seat belt to minimize shoulder discomfort
- A sheepskin steering wheel cover to protect hand joints by allowing a looser grip
- A portable step to help you get into an SUV or minivan
- A footrest to ease hip pain

Other tips for car travel:

- Make as many stops as necessary to avoid fatigue and to stretch when your joints start to feel stiff.

- At stoplights do exercises such as shoulder rolls, head tilts and neck stretches.
- Install special wide-angle side and rearview mirrors to increase your field of view without having to twist and turn in the driver's seat.
- If you don't think your car will be comfortable for your drive, consider renting a car that is. If you need suggestions, visit the Arthritis Foundation Web site (*www.arthritis.org*) for information about arthritis-friendly cars.
- Get someone to share the driving with you.

Think about . . .
planning my trip

For my next trip I'd love to travel to: _____

_____

_____

I'll need to find out these things about my desti-
nation to see if I can manage with my arthritis:

_____

_____

Potential problems that might arise from traveling to this place are: _____

_____

_____

Possible solutions are: _____

_____

_____

Resources

Centers for Disease Control and Prevention
To learn more about arthritis visit the CDC Web site at
www.cdc.gov/arthritis.

**National Institute of Arthritis and Musculoskeletal
and Skin Diseases**
Information Clearinghouse
National Institues of Health
1 AMS Circle
Bethesda, MD 20892-3675
Phone: 877-226-4267
www.niams.nih.gov

National Institutes of Health
Bldg. 31, Room 4C02
31 Center Dr.—MSC 2350
Bethesda, MD 20892-2350
Phone: 301-496-8190
www.nih.gov

American College of Rheumatology
1800 Century Place, Suite 250
Atlanta, GA 30345-4300
Phone: 404-633-3777
www.rheumatology.org

The American Occupational Therapy Association
4720 Montgomery Lane
P.O. Box 31220
Bethesda, MD 20824-1220
Phone: 301-652-2682
www.aota.org

Americans with Disabilities Act
www.ada.gov

The Arthritis Foundation

The mission of the Arthritis Foundation is to improve lives through leadership in the prevention, control and cure of arthritis and related diseases.

The Arthritis Foundation supports research with the greatest potential for advances and has invested more than $320 million in these efforts since its inception in 1948. Additionally, the Arthritis Foundation supports key public policy and advocacy efforts at a local and national level in order to make a difference on behalf of 70 million people living with arthritis. As your partner in taking greater control of arthritis, the Arthritis Foundation also offers a large number of programs and services nationwide to make life with arthritis easier and less painful and to help you become an active partner in your own health care. Contact us at (800) 283-7800 or visit us on the Web at *www.arthritis.org* to become an Arthritis Advocate or to find out how you can become involved.

Who Is Jack Canfield,
Cocreator of *Chicken Soup for the Soul*®?

Jack Canfield is one of America's leading experts in the development of human potential and personal effectiveness. He is both a dynamic, entertaining speaker and a highly sought-after trainer. Jack has a wonderful ability to inform and inspire audiences toward increased levels of self-esteem and peak performance. He has authored or coauthored numerous books, including *Dare to Win, The Aladdin Factor, 100 Ways to Build Self-Concept in the Classroom, Heart at Work* and *The Power of Focus.* His latest book is *The Success Principles.*

www.jackcanfield.com

Who Is Mark Victor Hansen,
Cocreator of *Chicken Soup for the Soul*®?

In the area of human potential, no one is more respected than **Mark Victor Hansen**. For more than thirty years, Mark has focused solely on helping people from all walks of life reshape their personal vision of what's possible. His powerful messages of possibility, opportunity and action have created powerful change in thousands of organizations and millions of individuals worldwide. He is a prolific writer of bestselling books such as *The One Minute*

Millionaire, The Power of Focus, The Aladdin Factor and *Dare to Win.*

www.markvictorhansen.com

Who Is David Pisetsky, MD., Ph.D.?

Dr. David Pisetsky is currently Professor of medicine and immunology and chief of rheumatology and immunology at the Duke University Medical Center. He received his M.D. and Ph.D. degrees from the Albert Einstein College of Medicine and then completed an internship and residency at the Yale-New Haven Hospital. After fellowship training at the National Institutes of Health, he joined the faculty of Duke. Dr. Pisetsky is an active clinician as well as researcher, investigating the mechansims of inflammation in rheumatoid arthritis and systemic lupus erythematosus. He has authored over 250 scientific articles and book chapters. From 2000 through 2005, he served as editor of *Arthritis and Rheumatism*, the leading journal in the field of rheumatology. In 2001, he received the Howley Prize from the Arthritis Foundation for his research.

Who Is Celia Slom Vimont?

Celia Slom Vimont is a health and medical writer. A graduate of the Columbia School of Journalism, she has written for magazines, newspapers and wire services for both consumers and physicians. The former director of editorial services for the American Lung Association, Celia served as in-house editor for books on asthma and smoking cessation for the association, and continues to write about a variety of lung health issues. She is the writer of three previous books in the *Chicken Soup Healthy Living* series: *Weight Loss, Menopause,* and *Asthma.* Celia lives in New York City with her husband and son.

More Chicken Soup

Many of the stories in this book were submitted by readers just like you. If you would like more information on submitting a story, visit our Web site at *www.chickensoup.com*. If you do not have Web access, we can also be reached at:

Chicken Soup for the Soul®
P.O. Box 30880, Santa Barbara, CA 93130
Fax: 805-563-2945

Contributors

Carolyn Dodge Adams was diagnosed with juvenile rheumatoid arthritis at the age of three. Today, she is a trainer and instructor for the Arthritis Foundation aquatic, exercise and self-help programs. Carolyn is dedicated to helping people with arthritis lead active and healthier lives.

Lawrence D. Elliott is a writer and has been an active Realtor® in Southern California for over seventeen years. His writing has been published both on the Internet and in print. He runs a network of real estate Web sites, which can be accessed through his main site at *www.LawrenceElliott.com*.

Linda Hanson, RRT-NPS, has worked for thirty years in most areas of respiratory care including intensive care units, neonatal, emergency rooms and in sleep labs. Her walking addiction started soon after she started work in pulmonary rehab. She is grateful for the lessons she learned from her patients.

Abha Iyengar lives in Delhi, India. She is a Kota Press Poetry Anthology Contest winner. Her work has appeared in *The Simple Touch of Fate, Knit Lit Too, Chicken Soup for the Healthy Soul, Moondance, Passing, Raven Chronicles, Gowanus Books, Writers against War,* among others. Her e-mail address is *abhaiyengar@rediffmail.com*.

Pamela Jenkins lives in Henryetta, Oklahoma, with her husband and four children. She is the office manager for a veterinary clinic. She has written stories for several *Chicken Soup for the Soul* books, *Country Magazine* and *Christian Woman*. E-mail Pamela at *calicoblessings@aol.com*.

Cindy La Ferle has successfully recovered from two hip replacement surgeries and is a nationally published essayist and newspaper columnist based in Royal Oak, Michigan. A new collection of her essays is published in *Writing Home* (Hearth Stone Books, 2005), which has earned several nonfiction awards and is a celebration of home, family and aging gracefully. Visit her Web site at *www.laferle.com*.

Rheumatoid arthritis forced **Fran McNabb** to take an early retirement from teaching, but she continued to find joy in words. Her first book, *Light in the Dark*, will be part of Avalon Books holiday lineup. The tender romance will be available in October 2006. Fran and her husband live on the Gulf Coast.

Eileen Valinoti's work has also appeared in *Chicken Soup for the Working Woman's Soul*.

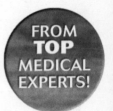